PHYSIO THERAPY DAD JOKES

- FROM PHYSIO MEMES -
IG: @PHYSIO_MEMES
WWW.PHYSIOMEMES.COM

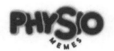

Table of Contents

DEDICATION

Dedicated to the Physio Memes #sQUAD that helps me push our mission forward to continue to grow the brand of the PT profession while Making Life Humerus. Without the team, we would not be able to make this book happen.

To all my coaches, friends, family, clients, and patients who have supported me in the non-traditional journey in my life and career.

There have been many times where I wanted to give up and go back on my vision and dreams to go back to the status quo and comfortable life, but you all are what helps me keep going.

Andrew Tran

Introduction

I am a physical therapist, and started what was originally a memes page for physical therapists on Instagram (@physio_memes) in 2016 a few months after I graduated from PT school at the University of Cincinnati. I was looking for a place that was consistently posting memes for Physios and couldn't find one, so I created one. My brain just thinks in memes so I created my own and share others that I find/get sent to me.

About a year later, I was looking for some shirts to wear for PTs, but the same thing happened. I couldn't find a website or company that sold PT swag. I started off creating my first shirt for a Thanksgiving Crossfit competition in 2017. It was a called the "Turkeys Get Up" which was a guy doing the Turkish Get Up, which is traditionally done with a kettle bell, but had the guy using a turkey. Someone saw the shirt I had, and asked where I got it from. I was so happy that someone else liked it! I couldn't hide the emotion, smirked, and told them that I made it. I sent them the link and made my first ever sale with a shirt.

I had plenty of ideas to put on shirts, just like I did with memes. I kept rolling my ideas out and ended up creating an entire apparel and products store for the physical therapy profession. Many of us in the PT profession know that most people don't know what we do. *"Can I get a massage?"*, *"Are you like a personal trainer?"*, *"Wait you have your doctorate?"*, and the list goes on. We all have been frustrated or wanted to roll our eyes when we hear statements like this.

While I was growing my page with memes and swag, I had a handful of people tell me I was helping brand the PT profession. I didn't realize it, but I was educating people in a different way with memes, jokes, punny apparel, and social media content that others could use to educate their patients with.

I know we have a long way to go with having people know exactly what we do, but I didn't want to be just another person that complained, and didn't do anything about it. This is my way of advocating for the profession.

Since then, my goal is to be able to help people grow their brands, which in turn helps each of us impact the lives of our family, friends, and community. We can't just sit around and wait for certain laws to pass, or have politicians vote a certain way. While this is helpful, we can all do our own part. We often educate patients once they are in our plan of care. What about those who do not come to us first?

When we can directly market so we can reach and educate our communities before they go get unnecessary injections, surgery and prescription opioids, that is where the true impact is.

Over the years, I have helped Pre-PTs, SPTs, PTs, and business owners on growing their brand, social media reach, and influence in their community.

This book is honestly just a fun project I have been thinking about doing over the last few years. I believe in spreading positivity, having fun during the journey, and bring you some laughter to #MakeLifeHumerus

The cringe-worthy PT Dad Jokes in this book are a compilation of jokes from our team and submissions from followers over the years.

Enjoy and submit any jokes, riddles, and stories to office@ physiomemes.com! We may use them for the next edition!

Section 1- Physical Therapy Dad Jokes

What did the snowman go to PT for?

Frozen Shoulder

———————————————

What did the mollusk say after a hard workout?

I've got a lot mussel fatigue.

What did the Clinical Instructor (CI) in the acute care setting say to the student when they asked "what do I need to get to help change this patient?"

Depends

What kind of jokes do optometrists tell?

Cornea ones

How do hippies usually
injure themselves?

Rolling their joints

Poop Jokes aren't my favorite, but do
you know where they rank?

Number 2

I don't trust people who dry needle.

They're all back stabbers.

———————————

You know, I used to work in a shoe
recycling store?

It was sole destroying.

I got my wife a prosthetic leg
for Christmas

It's not her main present, just a
stocking filler.

Do you know what happens if you get a
bladder infection?

Urine Trouble

Do you know the best way to a man's heart?

Between his 4th and 5th rib.

Which blood vessel won the talent show

The Jugular Vein

What's a urologists' favorite keyboard shortcut?

Control (cntrl) P

What did the dorsal column medial lemniscus say during therapy?

I had a lot of feelings

What did the PT say to the patient
who had a complete SCI that
started walking?

I can't believe you even had the nerve!

―――――――――

Why did the pillow go to the doctor?

He was feeling all stuffed up!

Where does a boat go when it's sick?

To the dock!

_____

Why did the PT lose his temper?

Because he didn't have any patients!

The patient kept telling me that they keep hearing a ringing sound.

I told them answer the phone!

Why aren't Physical Therapists allowed to start bar tabs at honkey-tonks?

Because PTs have been manipulating joints for years...

My patient told me that they broke their
leg in four places!

I told them "well, don't go back to
any of them!

———————————————

What did the PT do to my back to
make me laugh?

They cracked me up

What did the surgeon say when he saw
a long line?

May I cut in?

What do you call a PT that loves
manipulations?

A crack addict.

I turn heads every time I go to work

Well it makes sense, I'm a PT.

———————————————

What do you call a PT grandmother
who does manipulations?

A Gram Cracker

Do you know what really
makes me smile?

Facial muscles

Why did the muscle miss class?

...because it wasn't a-tendon!

Why did the bodybuilder borrow
a dictionary?

Because he wanted to know how to
define muscle.

What type of surgery did the
deli meat get?

A Bologna Amputation (BKA)

What muscle do you use to clean
a lightbulb?

The bulbospongiosis

———————————————————

What body part plays the best music?

The Iliotibial BAND

Have you seen the new show about connective tissue?

It's pretty fascia-nating

———————————————

What did the PT student say when they were practicing manual therapy in their cold classroom?

Manips Are Hard

Why did the patient keep asking for so much help for his patella femoral pain?

They were very knee-dy

What's the difference between a male and a female?

There's a Vas Deferens

What is a PTs favorite animal?

An Alli-GAIT-or

———————

What did the criminal die from when
the police officer locked him up?

Cardiac Arrest

I got fired from the bank the other day.
An old lady came in and asked me to
check her balance.

So I pushed her over.

Do you know all my of my boys want to
be valets when they grow up?

It's the biggest case of Parking Son's
I've ever seen.

Do you know you can hear the blood in your veins?

You just have to listen varicosely.

Did you know that dogs can't operate an MRI machine?

But Catscan

Do you know what gets on my nerves?

Myelin

―――――――――――――

What did one tonsil say to the
other tonsil?

I hear the doctor is taking us
out tonight!

Did you hear the jokes about the germ?

Never mind, I don't want to
spread it around

What did the dead pulmonologist say
to the other dead pulmonologist in
the graveyard?

Quit Coffin

Do want my old copies of Physical Therapy Monthly?

I've got loads of back issues.

Why did the Physical Therapist go bankrupt?

He owed too much in back taxes

After getting dry needled, my muscle pain is completely gone.

The pin really is mightier than the sore.

What did the winner of the muscle loss competition get?

A-trophy

My friend was complaining about my lack of muscle growth after being in the gym for 6 months...

I told him: "No whey!"

What has no legs but can do a split?

A banana.

Where does Muscle Milk come from?

Muscle mammary

———————————————

What do you call a girl who only likes
guys with big muscles?

A Biceptual

"How does a fork get a firmer body?"

"Utensil your muscles"

———————

What do you call a group of
bodybuilding priests at the gym?

A Muscle Mass

My PT told me to do 50
bodyweight squats…

…but I could barely do 20. And now
everyone in the morgue is staring at me.

———————————

Why did the PT break up with
his girlfriend?

She just wasn't working out.

Why was the PT so busy?

He had back to back meetings

What exercises did the Physio give
the engineer?

Bridges

What exercises did the PT
give the farmer?

Calf Raises

What do you say when you
go to a dinner with a bunch of
Physical Therapists?

Bone appetit!

My patient told me that they broke their leg in four places!

I told them "well, don't go back to any of them!

———————————

What's a ghost's favorite exercise?

Deadlifts

What kind of shoes do frogs wear?

Open Toad

What muscle group is most likely
to go to jail?

The Abductors

What did one sassy foot say to the other sassy foot?

Toe-tally

What muscle group is best at math?

The Adductors

A woman in labor suddenly shouted, "Shouldn't! Wouldn't! Couldn't! Didn't! Can't!

"Don't Worry," said the Doc. Those are just Contractions

Are you having trouble dropping kids off at the Super Bowl?

You may need to see a Pelvic PT.

What do you call an e-visit
for knee pain?

Patella Health

Where do you take someone who has
been injured in a Peek-a-Boo accident?

To the I.C.U

How do Pelvic Health PT's like their
eggs cooked?

Ovar-easy

Knock, knock?
Who's there?
HIPAA?
HIPAA Who?

Sorry, I can't tell you that

Why don't ants get sick?

They have little anty-bodies.

I took on a pelvic floor rotation and I've been able to see lots of different patients. Didn't even think I might be treating people with coccydynia though.

It's a pain in the ass.

A gingerbread man walks into the clinic
and complains that his knee hurts.

The PT says, have you tried icing it?

———————————————

What diagnosis did the mathematician
tell his patient?

"I'm sorry sir, you've had a
myocardial infraction"

What did the optimistic PT tell themselves every morning?

It's going tibia good day

"Before physical therapy, I was pain in the neck" - Pinched Nerve

Physical therapy puns are so…

Core-Knee.

I put my gait belt up on your hip.

When I lift, you lift, we lift.

Section 2: Humerus Ske-LOL-Tons

What do you call a funny bone?

A humerus.

They say there are two types of
PT professors:

One is humerus, but the other is
very sternum.

What's a skeleton's favorite instrument?

Trom-bone.

Why are skeletons so good at
chopping down trees?

They're LUMBARjacks!

How do you know if a spine
finds you funny?

It starts cracking up.

―――――――――――

What do you call two PTs who've got
each other's backs?

Vertebros

What do you call an alligator showing off his spine flexibility on the internet?

E-Reptile Disc Function

———————————————————

What do you call a piece of bread with no spine?

An invertebread

Where did the wrist bones drive
on the road?

In the Carpal Lane

———————————————————

How do two skeletons have sex?

They bone each other.

What do you call a skeleton who went
out in the snow?

A numb skull

———————————

What does a skeleton tile his roof with?

SHINgles!

What do you call it when a skeleton is having a great time?

An osteoblast.

What's the coolest part of a skeleton?

The hip.

What's the saddest movement in
the human body?

Scapular depression

Why was the skeleton so lonely?

He had no body

What do you call an angry patient
when the PT dry needles him in the
wrong muscle?

Triggered

What did the angry foot say when it
got amputated?

He Toe-d them off

I broke my finger the other day.

But on the other hand, I'm Okay.

———————————

What human body part is long, hard, bendable, and contains the letters P-E-N-S-I?

Your spine.

What do you call an Egyptian spine manipulator?

A Cairo-practor

Where do you learn about bones?

Osteoclasst.

Why does a skeleton always
tell the truth?

He wants tib-ia honest.

Why did the skeleton start a fight?

He had a bone to pick.

Which body part can help you find gold?

Leprecondyle

———————————

What do you call a person missing 75%
of their spine?

A quarter back.

Why are bones so calm?

Nothing gets under their skin.

What did the physical therapist bring to the potluck?

Spare ribs.

Why do skeletons get sick
on windy days?

It goes right through them.

Where do you imprison a
naughty skeleton?

A rib cage.

Why can't a group of skeletons ever get anything done?

It's a skeleton crew.

Did you hear about the skeleton that was almost picked apart by a group of wild dogs?

He marrowly escaped.

What do you call it when a skeleton is
having a great time?

An osteoblast.

Why can't a legless skeleton win
an argument?

They don't have a leg to stand on.

The right knee was telling the left knee jokes. After the right knee was done, what did the left knee say?

Patella Me More!

What did the doctor tell the skeleton who wanted to donate his body to science?

Spine on the dotted line.

What do you call a skeleton who lies?

A phoney-ba-boney.

What did the skeleton say when he proposed to his girlfriend?

Will you marrow me?

How do skeleton's get their
mail delivered?

By the bony express.

———————————

Why are skeletons such bad liars?

Everyone can see right through them.

What's a skeleton's favorite plant?

A BONE-zai tree. But if they don't like
that one, how about a S-pine tree?

How did the skeleton know it was going
to rain on Halloween?

He could feel it in his bones!

The skeleton canceled the gallery showing of his skull-ptures because his heart wasn't in it.

The skeleton played a melodic solo riff on his shiny sax-a-bone.

Did you hear about the skeleton that dropped out of PT school?

He just didn't have the stomach for it.

The skeleton cried his eyes out because he didn't have anybody to love.

What happened to the skeleton who stayed by the fire for too long?

He became bone dry

Skeleton 1: Why are graveyards so noisy?

Skeleton 2: I don't know. Why?

Skeleton 1: Because of all the coffin.

The skeleton didn't like to talk on the rotary skelephone

He preferred his cell bone.

What did the skeleton say while riding his Harley Davidson motorcycle?

I'm bone to be wild!

If you boil a funny bone it becomes a laughing stock.

That's humerus

Section 3: Skel-Lebrities

What happened to the guy who called
Terry Crews' muscles too small?

He died of dissing terry

Who was the most famous
skeleton detective?

Sherlock Bones

Who is the most famous historical ruler
of skeletons?

Napoleon Bone-a-part.

———————————

What is the most famous art piece
by a skeleton?

The Bona Lisa

Which skeleton is the most famous
motivational speaker?

Bony Robbins

Who is a skeleton's favorite actress?

Ulna Thurman

Who won the first season of
Skeleton Idol?

Skelly Clarkson

Did you hear who was in the lead to win
the skel-ection this year?

Skullary Clinton

What happened when Christopher Walken got bit by a zombie?

He became Christopher Walken Dead

Section 4: Skele-Tunes

What does Akon say when
he dies alone?

♪I am BONELY♪

What part of the body did the PT fix
when Eminem came in?

♪ *Shady's back* ♪

What is a Pediatric PTs
favorite rap song?

♪Baby, got back♪

━━━━━━━━━━━━━━━━━━━━━

How does Ice Cube cue his patients who
were struggling on his exercises?

♪You can do it, put your back into ♪

Section 5: PT Pick Up Lines

Hey girl, I've got a crutch on you.

———————

Are you adductor longus?

Because I'd like to ADD you to my life

You are such a QT.

Do you know what muscle is responsible for lateral rotation of my neck?

Your gluteus maximus

I aorta tell you how much I love you.

———————————

I ulna want to be with you

You make my heart have PVCs.

Hey are you Brocha's Aphasia?

Because you leave me speechless

Are you a coronary artery?

Because you are wrapped
around my heart

———————————————

I'm not checking you out

I'm analyzing your gait

Are you a pleural effusion?

Because I can't breathe around you

———————————————

Hey girl, ICU in my dreams.

Can I take your temperature?

You're looking hot today.

Wanna go study some anatomy?

Are you drowning?

Because I'm feeling the urge to give you CPR.

Are you COPD?

Because you take my breath away.

I didn't plan on specializing, but you seem pretty special to me.

I hope someday to be your emergency contact.

Are you a positive L3 myotome?

Cause you make my knees weak.

―――――――――

Can you check my dermatomes?

I seem to have lost my senses over you.

Are you responsible for discharging?

Cause I want you to check me out.

———————————————

Are you a transfer belt?

Cause you make me feel safe.

Excuse me, are you osteoporosis?

Because you're giving me a serious
bone condition!

Is that a reflex hammer in your pocket?

Or are you just happy to see me!

If I was an endoplasmic reticulum, how would you want me?

Smooth or rough? ;)

If I were an enzyme, I'd be
DNA helicase:

So I could unzip your genes!!

Are you a pulmonary embolus?

Because you take my breath away

Are you an incentive spirometer?

Cause I'm going to suck on
you every hour

What did the PT tell his crush at the Christmas party?

Kiss me under the mistle-toe

Girl are you Vitamin D?

Cause you make my bone hard

CONCLUSION: What's next?

Physio Memes, LLC

Follow us on social media to stay up-to-date on new releases with books, apparel, products, memes, and

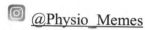 @Physio_Memes

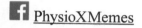 PhysioXMemes

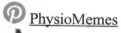 PhysioMemes

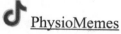 PhysioMemes

🖺 www.PhysioMemes.com for PT, PTA, SPT, SPTA apparel and products.

While we love to have fun providing memes and funny PT apparel, we also help businesses with growing their online brand. We teach you how to turn your followers into paying clients without using ads.

You can reach out for more information by emailing me at **Andrew@ physiomemes.com** with the subject line: "Business Branding".

Here is a free resource to set your Instagram profile up like a business card to increase the leads for your page:

engagingcontentkit.com/ideal-ig-profile

Thank you to **Jeremy Sutton** the #BookBoss for helping me take action to finally write this book. Thank you to **Christine Boucher** for helping make the silly edits that I missed. Thank you to **Naureen Imam** for the wonderful book cover!

Made in United States
Troutdale, OR
12/02/2024